T0120960

In the Shadow of
the Eclipse

In the Shadow of the Eclipse

Vivian R. Treves

iUniverse, Inc.
New York Lincoln Shanghai

In the Shadow of the Eclipse

Copyright © 2007 by Vivian R. Treves

All rights reserved. No part of this book may be used or reproduced by any means, graphic, electronic, or mechanical, including photocopying, recording, taping or by any information storage retrieval system without the written permission of the publisher except in the case of brief quotations embodied in critical articles and reviews.

iUniverse books may be ordered through booksellers or by contacting:

iUniverse
2021 Pine Lake Road, Suite 100
Lincoln, NE 68512
www.iuniverse.com
1-800-Authors (1-800-288-4677)

Because of the dynamic nature of the Internet, any Web addresses or links contained in this book may have changed since publication and may no longer be valid.

The views expressed in this work are solely those of the author and do not necessarily reflect the views of the publisher, and the publisher hereby disclaims any responsibility for them.

ISBN: 978-0-595-46369-5 (pbk)
ISBN: 978-0-595-90661-1 (ebk)

Printed in the United States of America

For those who suffer in silence
For those who search for the answers
For those who believe

Contents

PREFACE

Everyone else is in movement
And I am standing still
You and you and you are moving on
And I am stuck in the quagmire
Of a mystery illness
Which binds me and holds me
And holds on to me firmly in its grip
Rooted-in what-
In pain, in fatigue, in solitude
I watch as the world rushes on
"I used to be one of you," I cry out
Alas now I am not
"When?" I ask
When will I be astride again?
A vortex of hurt lashes at me
I know it will subside
And perhaps for a moment
I will live with peace of mind

DISMANTLING A LIFE

When I really think about it
I do remember feeling
My body breaking down
I don't exactly recall
When it was
But there was an exact time
I felt the meltdown
I felt something inside
Cracking up
And the machinery going awry
Something within had had enough
It could no longer take it
There was a flat out rebellion
A long term strike
Long overdue
Still to be resolved.

At first
I did not know why
I could not manage anymore
The myriad tasks
Which once were so easy to perform
I did not know why
My mind
My precious mind
Which functioned like a steel trap
Which worked like a perfectly oiled machine
Which was compared to a computer
That same mind
Simply did not compute anymore
I did not know why
I could no longer make it through
Those lengthy days and nights
In constant activity and motion
The machinery had never failed before
Could it be age?
Not possible
What were these ailments?
These signs of illness
Which one by one and over lapping one another
Brought me pain
Intermittently at first
Then gained strength
And visited for longer periods
With urgency
Demanding my attention
And finally swallowing whole
All my energy?

Getting a diagnosis
Not so easy
Let's eliminate
Eliminate what
All those other illnesses
One by one
MS
Lupus
Lyme
TB
No. No. No. No.
Depression
No. It is not DEPRESSION
This is physical
You must believe
Skeptical MD's
No cure
It can't be real
Non-Quantifiable symptoms
It doesn't exist
What do you mean??
It doesn't exist
There are just too many
Of us out there
With all those symptoms
The same symptoms
Hasn't anyone noticed
The numbers lately?
Don't blame those MD's
It's much easier to ignore us

There is a gaping
Wound in my soul
And no needle and thread
To repair it

Pain has been oozing out
For sometime
First in silence
Then with tears
Floods of words

Then the pain bellowed
Before retreating
To just being
An enormous open wound

Having been unable
To find
The right needle and thread
To close it up

This is just a world of initials
CFS, CFIDS, EBV, HHV 6
No causes
No cures
A lot of maybes
No sure fire yes
It exists, it doesn't
Who says?
Have you tried being
A victim/patient lately?

Why is it
That everyone seems
To know someone
Who has this illness
And yet many know so little
Nor seem to really get it
Nor seem to take it seriously
After all
We are not scarred
Maimed, moribund
On the outside at least
So I guess they guess
We're really okay
But we are not.

My mind wanders in a strange world
That is neither here nor there
Not awake, yet not asleep
Somewhere up there
In between
Thoughts roam freely
Sometimes in anger
Sometimes carefree
And yet I am
A prisoner of this place
Unable to leave
At my command.

The notion of time
Has changed of late

Life used to be played
In fast forward time
Until the mechanisms
Unraveled

It seems for now
They cannot be fixed

So the light and dark
Trade places in slow motion

All that went by in a blur
Is now in sharp focus
Close up
Detailed
What was in the background
Is in the foreground
It is a new way of
Seeing
Hearing
In slo mo
A different notion of living.

Having CFS
Is like
Belonging to a club
You don't want to
Be a member of
The members themselves
Are wonderful
Kind. Generous. Empathetic.
They don't want to belong either
But it is nice
To find comfort in misery
And know we are not alone.

It is as if
A violent storm
Enters my brain
And wreaks havoc
On all the senses

The system shuts down
In pain.
The eyes close
Tight.
The body is prone,
Immobile.

And there is nothing to be done
Until the storm passes.

The voices in the waiting room
Speak from pain and uncertainty
The voices in the waiting room
Are eager to share their experiences
They want confirmation
That they are not alone with this suffering

The voices in the waiting room
Echo one another
Which cures have you tried?
How badly are you feeling?
Are you as disabled as I am?
They won't give you disability?
You have to sell your home?
You're moving back in with your family?
You have no one?
The brain fog, the headaches, the fevers
The need to rest, rest, rest

The voices in the waiting room
Change from week to week
But the chorus grows louder
It rebounds from the walls
Crying to be heard out there, in the world
Why do they come week after week to the waiting room?
Perhaps they come to exercise their voices
And to share in the hope of imminent recovery

DETAINED IN EXILE

Today is a bad CFS day
Today is the kind of day
I cannot get my head off the pillow
Today is the kind of day
It is an effort to turn over
And I wish someone was here
To cook and serve me a meal
Although I do not really have the strength
To even chew the food
Today is the kind of day
Where every gesture costs me
I do not even have the strength
To speak
Although there is dialogue in my brain
And the words acknowledge
I do not have the strength
And I suffer
Even though I have learned
To play by the rules.
There is nothing to do
I must follow
What the disease dictates
It rules me
I do not rule it
Notwithstanding that, at first
I thought I was superwoman
I have since learned
I am not.

I am but a
Muted version of
My former self
The trademark vibrancy
Is but a memory
The sharp colors of my life
Replaced by drab ones
The clarity of mind
Softened around the edges
The focus unpredictable

Yesterday
For a brief while
I felt normal
I felt like the old me
What a strange sensation
It was like meeting
An old friend
Someone I had not
Seen for a long time
What a pleasant visit we had
But it did not last long.

Having CFS
Is kind of like
Having a prison sentence
A unique prison it is
Though. Yes,
The body is confined
To the vicissitudes
Of the day, hour and minute
But the mind-
It is free to wander
Far and wide
To explore abandoned
Channels of the soul
To examine long forgotten
And long lost episodes
In the chapters of life

Sometime CFS
Plays tricks on the mind
It alters our perceptions
It challenges our memories
But it cannot
Follow us
Down the dark
And luminous pathways
Of our soul
It cannot contain
The longing for the answers
It cannot stop
The heart from beating.

Guess we will never know
Will we?
What paths we would have
Could have taken
Prior to the illness
What glory what success
What pain what failure
We'll never know will we?
Silly to even think about it
Those are no longer options
Are they?
Should we be even wondering?
Probably not.
It's hard enough
To deal with today
And not sigh

I cannot see me
The way you see me
I cannot see beyond the illness
Often I am just the disease
There is no me
And the symptoms are
My definition
You see what looks like
A healthy person
No scars, no casts,
No visible signs
You only hear my words
It is impossible to image
Losing oneself
To a misnamed state of being

Now that the brain fog has lifted
And I eat the right food
The available minutes
Have turned into
A few hours a day
A few hours to clearly
Get a few things done.
No time for bullshit
Every breath is accounted for
Every gesture is weighed
No room for waste
No fat to trim
It's just the way it is
Actually it's amazing
What one can accomplish in three hours
When one is focused
Oh, well. Time is up.
Already. Oh well.
There is tomorrow to look forward to
If you play by the rules

Before there was the sound
Of music and laughter
Of applause and the clinking
Of glasses in crowded spaces

Now there are waves of silence
Ringing in my ear
For only in the quiet
Is it possible to think
To avoid the confusion
Of babbling voices
The pressure to respond
To impossible situations

The silence is vast
The waves go in and out like the tide
The silence is dark, the silence is light
And yet its constant companionship is comforting

In the dark
It wraps me like a blanket protecting the night
In the daylight
It sparkles and heals the soul
Awesome it is this silence
Unlike the one of the past
Which haunted the loneliness in my soul.

Sometimes
I find it difficult
To contain the grief
The overwhelming
And profound sadness
Which knows no depth
Which burrows in
My soul for so long
I cannot remember
When it took possession
When it altered the
Course of my life
I do try to keep it down
But sometimes
It just escapes.

We are truly and only
A vast worldwide cacophony of
Voices in a waiting room
Stuck in a medical vacuum
Our illness is misnamed
The few doctors who believe
Are but sleuths in a vast mystery universe
Ill heeded by the uninterested majority of MD's

So we sit and wait
Faceless, nameless
Bursting with the feeble energy
We can muster up on a good day
How can the rest of you understand?
We look so good and feel so bad
When we are lying down mute in pain
You are not there to watch
You only hear about it perhaps
And if it sinks in you say you envy us
You wish you too could take a nap
Not this one- - - -believe us
Our immune system does not know the time of day
It is just on- - - -eternally it seems
And we exist askew of all of you
Hoping for a few good moments, hours, days
And the pain is just constant, unbearable
Lots of you tune out, walk away
It and we are just too boring, non-existent
We should have checked you off long ago anyway

There are higher planes of existence
And there we wait and learn.

On sunnier days
The challenges
Become gifts of wonder
To behold
As they sparkle and bedazzle
They seem imminently
Within our grasp
They create a sense of excitement
Of bold adventure yet to be realized
The gifts are there for the taking
If we only find the strength within
To meet the challenges head-on
And not to look back at what we leave behind
The comfort of the old ways, the old friends,
The persona we used to inhabit
Who by virtue of this circumstance
No longer can be
Only by shedding those guises
Are the gifts being offered
Those bright shiny objects of desire
Attainable

Is the immune system connected to the soul
Or is the soul connected to the immune system?
Why is it that when the immune system breaks down
The soul system appears to reveal its inner workings
It was always there albeit in hiding it seems
Why does it open its door so wide
That we are forced to step in and examine ourselves
When we had that opportunity long ago
And chose to ignore that treasure
Which was so easily within our grasp
As we reached for lesser riches out there
Out there where the souls carries little value
And what is treasured is of such meager import
And yet it often blinds us
Until one day our immunity is shattered
And by consequence embers are ignited
Embers of a previously moribund soul system

I am taking my illness with me to the sea
Yes it is coming on vacation too
And together we will sit on the shore
And contemplate the waves
And listen to the constant lapping of the water
And wonder about the tides

And I will wish
Will wish
That I could take this illness
And put it in a bottle
And seal it
And send it off shore
Never to be heard from again

The Joys of the Day

It is easier to be happy now
For the joys are little ones
Not having a headache
Or a muscle ache
Or forgetting something
Noticing that the sun is shining
Listening to hear birds singing
Sleeping the whole night fitfully
Having a friend call
Knowing that today
I am better than yesterday
These are the little joys.

LIVING IN THE SHADOW OF THE ECLIPSE

We live in the shadow of the eclipse
Which has darkened our lives
And we wonder when it will move on
Allowing the light to shine once again in our lives
The eclipse has altered our state
Turning us into shadow people
It has bought us pain and sorrow and sadness
We have had to charge up our inner brightness
To bring about the daily healing
We need to survive

The good thing about eclipses
Is that they move on
And then we shall be whole again

I cannot remember
What it feels like to be well
I cannot remember
Waking up in the morning
And knowing what it is like being well
I cannot remember
When I last looked in the mirror
And actually saw me
The person in the mirror now
Is just a shadow
A poor reflection
Of a once active thriving being
Where did I go?
I didn't even have a chance to say
Good-bye
I just disappeared
And in my place
Is a pallid version of a lost being
A being who waits patiently
For the colors to come back
Into her life

In the silence
I can hear the sound of tears
Falling loud and hard
The tears of loss and frustration
The tears of anger
That no one is listening
Or paying attention
Or rather they are deriding
Our incomprehensible demise

In the dark
I can see well now and focus
As if a light were shining on them
I can focus
On all the wrongs which were....
And I could not even see them then
So close they were before me

Yes this illness
Has taken so much away
And the road to recovery is slow
But one thing is clear
Things will never be the same
They will undoubtedly be better
For this new night vision
Has forged a path, has moved the ills aside
Has isolated the real problems

Yes the darkness has given way to light
And never more will we accept less
Life can only be better.

The more life is removed from me
The more I become addicted to it
I savor it
I lust for it
And right now I cannot live it
I am forced to watch and observe
From the sidelines

Once in awhile
For a few hours at a time
I am allowed to play
And make a few points
How I savor these moments
And wish I could be in the game full time

My thoughts
Are like whirling dervishes
As they gallop wantonly
Across the landscape of my brain
They whirl on and on
Try as I might to calm them down
The illness will not allow them to stop

Though I am exhausted
My mind rushes from thought to thought
My body and soul yearn for sleep
As the pattern repeats itself each night
The sleep will not come
Until pure exhaustion wins over
And for a brief while
There is respite

Days of the calendar
No longer count
Months and seasons
Have but little import
What really have importance
Are the hours
One is functional
The hours
One can do and be
The hours
One can have a decent conversation
One can write a check
Take care of business
Make a meal
Keep the home clean
How quickly these moments go by
How fast the good times
Before it becomes the minutes
To breakdown
The minutes left
To naptime
To bedtime
To turn off
Nothing to be done
That is how time is marked
In the world of CFIDS.

Living with CFIDS
Is like living in a dream world
Where thoughts float by like cumulous clouds
They are no longer anchored the way they used to be
These thoughts are haphazard and wild
They have no direction
The computer which was the brain
Is definitely on the fritz
It has a virus which is oh so mischievous
One can simply no longer count on one's mind
It is on. It is off. It wanders.
Some days some parts work just fine
Then they just fail. No explanation given
No future promises or working right
It is just so hard to adjust
It is just so hard to be still
And not wonder
When all the pieces will be functional.

If you approach the shadow of the eclipse
And stand near and listen and observe
You can see us clearly in pain
And
You may hear us calling out
Imploring you to listen

We are the shadow people
We did not ask to become so
It simply happened and here we are
And we beg you to listen and learn with us
While we wait for the eclipse to move on
And return the light into our lives.

AFTERWARD

The illness succeeded in tearing me
Wide open to the core
The hollow exterior shed
Exposing the deeply planted roots
Of my soul
For all to see
And yet it could not uproot me
For I was quite solid
And remain to this day unbroken
Like an aged tree
Whose gnarled roots are embedded
Deep deep into the soil
Where the core is immutable locked in forever
Now it is time for a new trunk
To cover over the exposure
And once again to blossom leaves
As the seasons turn

978-0-595-46369-5
0-595-46369-X

Printed in the United States
By Bookmasters